THE DOPAMINE NUTRITION DIET COOKBOOK

DR JULIET HENRY

INTRODUCTION

Dopamine is a crucial neurotransmitter, often referred to as the "feel-good" or "reward" neurotransmitter due to its involvement in various aspects of mood regulation, pleasure, and motivation. It plays a pivotal role in the central nervous system, serving as a chemical messenger that facilitates communication between nerve cells, or neurons, in the brain. Understanding the intricacies of dopamine is essential for grasping the core principles of the Dopamine Nutrition Diet Cookbook.

The Nature of Dopamine:

Definition: Dopamine is a monoamine neurotransmitter, belonging to the catecholamine family, and is synthesized from the amino acid tyrosine. It functions both as a neurotransmitter and a precursor to other essential neurotransmitters, making it indispensable for overall neurological health.

Neurotransmission: Dopamine is synthesized in specific regions of the brain, primarily within the substantia nigra and the ventral tegmental area. Once produced, it travels across synapses, the junctions between nerve cells, to transmit signals from one neuron to another. This transmission is a fundamental process in various cognitive and emotional functions.

Dopamine and Mood Regulation:

Reward Pathway: Dopamine is intricately linked to the brain's reward system, influencing feelings of pleasure and reinforcement. Activities such as eating, socializing, and achieving goals trigger the release of dopamine, creating a sense of reward and motivation.

Mood and Emotion: Dopamine also plays a crucial role in regulating mood and emotions. Imbalances in dopamine levels have been associated with conditions like depression, anxiety, and other mood disorders. Understanding how nutrition impacts dopamine production is a key aspect of the Dopamine Nutrition Diet Cookbook.

Nutrition and Dopamine

Precursor to Dopamine: Tyrosine, an amino acid found in various foods, serves as the precursor to dopamine. The Dopamine Nutrition Diet Cookbook focuses on incorporating tyrosine-rich foods to support the body's natural production of dopamine.

Nutrients and Cofactors: Beyond tyrosine, certain vitamins and minerals, such as vitamin B6, folate, and iron, act as cofactors in the synthesis of dopamine. The cookbook emphasizes the importance of a well-balanced diet that provides these essential nutrients for optimal dopamine function.

In essence, dopamine is a multifaceted neurotransmitter with profound implications for mental and emotional well-being. The Dopamine Nutrition Diet Cookbook endeavors to elucidate the connection between nutrition, dopamine production, and overall health, offering a comprehensive guide to harnessing the benefits of dopamine-boosting foods in a delicious and nourishing way.

THE IMPORTANCE OF DOPAMINE

Reward and Pleasure: Dopamine is often referred to as the brain's "feel-good" neurotransmitter because it is involved in the brain's reward system. It plays a key role in reinforcing behaviors that are essential for survival, such as eating, drinking, and reproduction. By experiencing pleasure and satisfaction from these activities, individuals are motivated to repeat them, ensuring the continuation of essential behaviors for survival.

Motivation and Goal-Oriented Behavior: Dopamine is closely linked to motivation and goal-directed behavior. It helps individuals anticipate rewards and take action to achieve them. Healthy dopamine levels are crucial for maintaining motivation, focus, and perseverance in pursuing goals, whether they are related to career, relationships, or personal development.

Cognitive Function: Dopamine also influences various cognitive functions, including attention, learning, memory, and decision-making. Optimal dopamine levels are essential for sustaining attention, processing information efficiently, forming memories, and making sound decisions. Imbalances in dopamine levels have been associated with cognitive impairments, such as difficulties in concentration, memory deficits, and impaired executive function.

Emotional Regulation: Dopamine plays a role in regulating emotions and mood. Adequate dopamine levels contribute to emotional stability, resilience to stress, and a positive outlook on life. Conversely, dysregulation of dopamine signaling has been implicated in mood disorders such as depression, anxiety, and addiction.

Motor Function: In addition to its role in cognitive and emotional processes, dopamine is crucial for controlling motor function and movement. It is produced in regions of the brain involved in motor control, including the substantia nigra and striatum. Dopamine deficiency in these areas can lead to motor symptoms characteristic of neurological disorders such as Parkinson's disease.

Understanding the importance of dopamine in brain function provides the framework for selecting and preparing foods that support optimal dopamine levels. By focusing on nutrient-dense ingredients known to enhance dopamine production and signaling, readers can potentially improve their mood, motivation, cognitive function, and overall well-being.

How Nutrition Affects Dopamine Levels:

Dopamine, often referred to as the "feel-good" neurotransmitter, plays a pivotal role in various aspects of cognitive and emotional functioning. Nutrition exerts a profound influence on dopamine levels through several mechanisms, impacting both its synthesis and activity within the brain.

1. Precursor Availability: Dopamine is synthesized from the amino acid tyrosine, which is obtained through dietary protein sources. Foods rich in tyrosine, such as poultry, fish, dairy products, nuts, seeds, and legumes, provide the necessary building blocks for dopamine production. In your

cookbook, you'll highlight recipes featuring these tyrosine-rich ingredients to support optimal dopamine synthesis.

2. Cofactors and Coenzymes: Certain vitamins and minerals serve as cofactors and coenzymes in the enzymatic pathways responsible for dopamine synthesis and metabolism. For instance, vitamin B6, folate, iron, magnesium, and zinc are essential for the conversion of tyrosine into dopamine. By incorporating foods abundant in these micronutrients, such as leafy greens, whole grains, lean meats, and seeds, your cookbook will facilitate the availability of these vital nutrients to support dopamine production.

3. Regulation of Dopamine Release: Nutritional factors can influence the release and reuptake of dopamine within the

synaptic cleft. For example, carbohydrates stimulate insulin release, which enhances the uptake of amino acids—including tyrosine—into cells, thereby promoting dopamine synthesis. Complex carbohydrates, found in whole grains, fruits, and vegetables, provide sustained energy and help maintain stable dopamine levels throughout the day.

4. Anti-inflammatory Properties: Chronic inflammation can impair dopamine signaling and contribute to neurodegenerative conditions like Parkinson's disease. By emphasizing an anti-inflammatory dietary pattern rich in antioxidants, omega-3 fatty acids, and phytonutrients, your cookbook can mitigate inflammation and preserve optimal dopamine function. Ingredients such as berries, fatty fish, turmeric, and green tea possess potent anti-inflammatory properties and can be incorporated into delicious recipes featured in your book.

5. Gut-Brain Axis: Emerging research suggests a bidirectional communication pathway between the gut and the brain, known as the gut-brain axis, which profoundly influences neurotransmitter function, including dopamine. A balanced and diverse diet that supports gut health, including probiotic-rich foods like yogurt, kefir, and fermented vegetables, may indirectly enhance dopamine production and mitigate symptoms of mood disorders.

The nutritional composition of one's diet significantly impacts dopamine levels and neurotransmitter function. By adopting a dietary approach that prioritizes dopamine-boosting foods, micronutrient-rich ingredients, and anti-inflammatory nutrients, individuals can optimize brain health, mood stability, and overall well-being.

CHAPTER ONE

Principles and Fundamentals:

Unveiling the core principles that underpin the Dopamine Nutrition Diet, this section delves into the scientific basis of dopamine's role in brain function and overall health.

Explaining how the diet revolves around optimizing the synthesis of dopamine through strategic food choices and nutrient intake.

Benefits of the Dopamine Nutrition Diet

Articulating the numerous advantages and positive effects associated with adopting the Dopamine Nutrition Diet, such as enhanced mood, improved cognitive function, and increased energy levels.

Providing evidence-based insights into the potential impact of dopamine-boosting foods on mental health and cognitive performance.

Dopamine-Boosting Foods and Nutrients

Enumerating a comprehensive list of foods rich in tyrosine, the precursor to dopamine, and elucidating their significance in supporting optimal dopamine production.

Detailing the role of essential vitamins, minerals, and other nutrients that play a crucial part in the synthesis and regulation of dopamine levels.

Integration with the Cookbook's Recipes:

Bridging the theoretical understanding of the Dopamine Nutrition Diet with practical application, this section seamlessly connects the exploration to the diverse and delicious recipes featured in the cookbook.

Demonstrating how each recipe aligns with the diet's principles, ensuring that readers can easily incorporate dopamine-boosting foods into their daily meals.

Long-Term Health and Lifestyle Implications:

Discussing the potential long-term benefits of embracing the Dopamine Nutrition Diet in terms of overall health, well-being, and disease prevention.

Offering insights into how sustained adherence to the diet may contribute to a balanced and dopamine-supported lifestyle.

"Foods Rich in Tyrosine: The Precursor to Dopamine" is a crucial chapter in "The Dopamine Nutrition Diet Cookbook," as it delves into the foundational understanding of how the amino acid tyrosine plays a pivotal role in the synthesis of dopamine, a neurotransmitter associated with mood regulation, motivation, and overall cognitive function. This chapter aims to educate readers on the significance of tyrosine as a precursor to dopamine production and provides comprehensive insights into incorporating tyrosine-rich foods into their diet.

HERBS AND SPICES FOR DOPAMINE

1. **Turmeric:** This vibrant spice contains curcumin, a compound with potent antioxidant and anti-inflammatory properties. Research suggests that curcumin may help increase dopamine levels in the brain by protecting dopamine-producing neurons from oxidative stress and inflammation.

2. **Saffron**: Known for its distinct aroma and flavor, saffron contains compounds like crocin and crocetin, which have been studied for their neuroprotective effects. Some studies indicate that saffron may help regulate dopamine levels and enhance mood, making it a valuable addition to dishes aimed at supporting brain health.

3. **Rosemary**: A fragrant herb commonly used in Mediterranean cuisine, rosemary contains rosmarinic acid and other compounds with antioxidant and anti-inflammatory properties. Research suggests that rosemary extract may help protect dopamine neurons from damage and support overall brain health.

4. **Basil:** With its fresh and aromatic flavor, basil is not only a popular culinary herb but also a source of essential nutrients and

bioactive compounds. Basil contains phytochemicals like eugenol and rosmarinic acid, which have been studied for their potential neuroprotective effects and ability to support dopamine function in the brain.

5. **Ginger:** Widely used in both savory and sweet dishes, ginger is prized for its unique flavor and medicinal properties. Ginger contains bioactive compounds like gingerol and shogaol, which possess antioxidant and anti-inflammatory properties. While research specifically linking ginger to dopamine levels is limited, its overall neuroprotective effects suggest it may indirectly support dopamine function.

6. **Cinnamon:** This sweet and aromatic spice is not only delicious but also rich in antioxidants and anti-inflammatory compounds. Studies have shown that

cinnamon may help improve insulin sensitivity and regulate blood sugar levels, which can indirectly influence dopamine production and neurotransmitter balance in the brain.

7. **Oregano:** A staple herb in Mediterranean cuisine, oregano contains potent antioxidants like rosmarinic acid and thymol. These compounds have been studied for their neuroprotective effects and potential to support dopamine function in the brain, although more research is needed to fully understand their mechanisms of action.

Incorporating these herbs and spices into recipes featured in your cookbook can not only enhance the flavor and aroma of dishes but also provide potential health benefits by supporting dopamine levels and overall brain health. Including a variety of herbs and spices in the diet is a delicious and practical way to promote optimal brain function and well-being as part of the Dopamine Nutrition Diet.

CHAPTER TWO

BREAKFAST RECIPES

Dopamine-Boosting Smoothie

Ingredients:

- 1 cup spinach

- 1/2 cup blueberries

- 1/2 banana

- 1 tablespoon almond butter

- 1/2 cup almond milk

- 1 teaspoon chia seeds

Instructions:

1. Blend all ingredients until smooth.

2. Pour into a glass and enjoy immediately.

Tyrosine-Rich Oatmeal

Ingredients:

- 1/2 cup rolled oats

- 1 cup water or almond milk

- 1/2 sliced banana

- 1 tablespoon walnuts, chopped

- 1 teaspoon honey or maple syrup

Instructions:

1. Cook oats according to package instructions.

2. Top with sliced banana, chopped walnuts, and drizzle with honey or maple syrup.

Dopamine-Boosting Breakfast Burrito

Ingredients:

- 2 eggs

- 1/4 cup black beans, drained and rinsed

- 2 tablespoons diced bell peppers

- 2 tablespoons diced tomatoes

- 2 tablespoons shredded cheddar cheese

- 2 whole grain tortillas

Instructions:

1. Scramble eggs in a pan until cooked.

2. Warm tortillas and fill with scrambled eggs, black beans, bell peppers, tomatoes, and cheese.

3. Roll up and serve hot.

Dopamine-Enhancing Chia Pudding

Ingredients:

- 2 tablespoons chia seeds

- 1/2 cup almond milk

- 1/2 teaspoon vanilla extract

- 1/2 cup mixed berries

Instructions:

1. Mix chia seeds, almond milk, and vanilla extract in a bowl.

2. Let sit in the refrigerator for at least 30 minutes or until thickened.

3. Top with mixed berries before serving.

] Dopamine-Boosting Yogurt Parfait

Ingredients:

- 1/2 cup Greek yogurt

- 1/4 cup granola

- 1/4 cup mixed berries

- 1 tablespoon honey

Instructions:

1. Layer Greek yogurt, granola, mixed berries, and honey in a glass.

2. Repeat layers as desired.

3. Serve chilled.

Dopamine-Packed Breakfast Sandwich

Ingredients:

- 2 slices whole grain bread

- 1 egg, fried or scrambled

- 1 slice avocado

- 1 slice tomato

- Salt and pepper to taste

Instructions:

1. Toast whole grain bread until golden brown.

2. Top one slice with fried or scrambled egg, avocado, tomato, salt, and pepper.

3. Place the other slice of bread on top to form a sandwich.

4. Serve warm.

Dopamine-Boosting Breakfast Bowl

Ingredients:

- 1/2 cup cooked quinoa

- 1/4 cup sliced almonds

- 1/4 cup diced mango

- 1/4 cup diced pineapple

- 1 tablespoon shredded coconut

Instructions:

1. Mix cooked quinoa, sliced almonds, diced mango, diced pineapple, and shredded coconut in a bowl.

2. Enjoy as is or drizzle with honey for added sweetness.

Dopamine-Enhancing Breakfast Wrap

Ingredients:

- 1 whole grain wrap

- 2 tablespoons almond butter

- 1/2 banana, sliced

- 1 tablespoon honey

- 1 tablespoon chia seeds

Instructions:

1. Spread almond butter evenly on the whole grain wrap.

2. Arrange sliced banana on top of the almond butter.

3. Drizzle with honey and sprinkle with chia seeds.

4. Roll up the wrap and slice in half before serving.

Dopamine-Boosting Breakfast Cookies

Ingredients:

- 1 cup rolled oats

- 1 ripe banana, mashed

- 1/4 cup almond butter

- 1/4 cup dark chocolate chips

- 1/4 cup chopped walnuts

Instructions:

1. Preheat oven to 350°F (175°C) and line a baking sheet with parchment paper.

2. In a bowl, combine rolled oats, mashed banana, almond butter, dark chocolate chips, and chopped walnuts until well mixed.

3. Scoop spoonfuls of the mixture onto the prepared baking sheet and flatten slightly with a fork.

4. Bake for 12-15 minutes or until golden brown.

5. Allow to cool before serving.

Dopamine-Boosting Breakfast Muffins

Ingredients:

- 1 cup almond flour

- 1/4 cup coconut flour

- 1 teaspoon baking powder

- 1/4 teaspoon salt

- 2 ripe bananas, mashed

- 2 eggs

- 1/4 cup almond milk

- 1/4 cup maple syrup

- 1 teaspoon vanilla extract

Instructions:

1. Preheat oven to 350°F (175°C) and line a muffin tin with paper liners.

2. In a large bowl, whisk together almond flour, coconut flour, baking powder, and salt.

3. In another bowl, mix mashed bananas, eggs, almond milk, maple syrup, and vanilla extract until well combined.

4. Gradually add wet ingredients to dry ingredients, stirring until just combined.

5. Divide batter evenly among muffin cups.

6. Bake for 20-25 minutes or until a toothpick inserted into the center comes out clean.

7. Allow muffins to cool before serving.

Dopamine-Boosting Acai Bowl

Ingredients:

- 1 packet frozen acai puree

- 1/2 banana, sliced

- 1/4 cup mixed berries

- 1/4 cup granola

- 1 tablespoon almond butter

- 1 teaspoon chia seeds

Instructions:

1. Blend frozen acai puree until smooth.

2. Pour blended acai into a bowl.

3. Top with sliced banana, mixed berries, granola, almond butter, and chia seeds.

4. Serve immediately.

Dopamine-Enhancing Shakshuka

Ingredients:

- 2 eggs

- 1/2 cup tomato sauce

- 1/4 cup diced bell peppers

- 1/4 cup diced onions

- 1 clove garlic, minced

- 1/2 teaspoon cumin

- Salt and pepper to taste

- Fresh parsley for garnish

Instructions:

1. Heat olive oil in a skillet over medium heat.

2. Add diced bell peppers, onions, and garlic. Cook until softened.

3. Stir in tomato sauce and cumin. Simmer for 5 minutes.

4. Create small wells in the sauce and crack eggs into them.

5. Cover and cook until eggs are set, about 5-7 minutes.

6. Season with salt and pepper.

7. Garnish with fresh parsley before serving.

13. Dopamine-Boosting Breakfast Quinoa Salad

Ingredients:

- 1 cup cooked quinoa

- 1/4 cup diced cucumber

- 1/4 cup diced tomatoes

- 2 tablespoons chopped fresh basil

- 2 tablespoons crumbled feta cheese

- 1 tablespoon extra virgin olive oil

- 1 tablespoon balsamic vinegar

- Salt and pepper to taste

Instructions:

1. In a bowl, combine cooked quinoa, diced cucumber, diced tomatoes, chopped fresh basil, and crumbled feta cheese.

2. Drizzle with extra virgin olive oil and balsamic vinegar.

3. Season with salt and pepper.

4. Toss gently to combine.

5. Serve chilled or at room temperature.

Dopamine-Enhancing Banana Pancakes

Ingredients:

- 1 ripe banana, mashed

- 2 eggs

- 1/4 teaspoon cinnamon

- 1/4 teaspoon vanilla extract

- Cooking spray or coconut oil for greasing

Instructions:

1. In a bowl, combine mashed banana, eggs, cinnamon, and vanilla extract. Mix until well combined.

2. Heat a skillet over medium heat and lightly grease with cooking spray or coconut oil.

3. Pour small portions of the batter onto the skillet to form pancakes.

4. Cook until bubbles form on the surface, then flip and cook until golden brown on the other side.

5. Serve warm with your favorite toppings such as fresh fruit, yogurt, or maple syrup.

Dopamine-Boosting Breakfast Pizza

Ingredients:

- 1 whole grain pita bread or flatbread

- 2 tablespoons marinara sauce

- 1/4 cup diced bell peppers

- 1/4 cup diced onions

- 1/4 cup sliced mushrooms

- 1/4 cup shredded mozzarella cheese

- 2 eggs

Instructions:

1. Preheat oven to 375°F (190°C).

2. Spread marinara sauce evenly over the pita bread.

3. Top with diced bell peppers, onions, mushrooms, and shredded mozzarella cheese.

4. Create two small wells in the toppings and crack eggs into them.

5. Bake for 10-12 minutes or until the egg whites are set and the cheese is melted.

6. Slice and serve hot.

Dopamine-Boosting Breakfast Tacos

Ingredients:

- 2 corn tortillas

- 2 eggs

- 1/4 cup black beans, drained and rinsed

- 1/4 avocado, sliced

- 2 tablespoons salsa

- Fresh cilantro for garnish

Instructions:

1. Heat corn tortillas in a skillet until warmed through.

2. Cook eggs to your preference (scrambled, fried, or poached).

3. Fill each tortilla with scrambled eggs, black beans, avocado slices, salsa, and garnish with fresh cilantro.

4. Serve immediately.

Dopamine-Enhancing Overnight Oats

Ingredients:

- 1/2 cup rolled oats

- 1/2 cup almond milk

- 1/4 cup Greek yogurt

- 1 tablespoon chia seeds

- 1 tablespoon honey or maple syrup

- 1/4 cup mixed berries

Instructions:

1. In a jar or container, combine rolled oats, almond milk, Greek yogurt, chia seeds, and honey or maple syrup. Stir well.

2. Cover and refrigerate overnight.

3. In the morning, top with mixed berries before serving.

Dopamine-Boosting Breakfast Sushi

Ingredients:

- 2 slices whole grain bread

- 2 tablespoons almond butter

- 1 banana, peeled

- 1 tablespoon honey

- 1 tablespoon unsweetened coconut flakes

Instructions:

1. Flatten bread slices with a rolling pin.

2. Spread almond butter evenly over each slice.

3. Place a peeled banana at one end of each bread slice and roll up tightly.

4. Slice each roll into bite-sized pieces.

5. Drizzle with honey and sprinkle with unsweetened coconut flakes.

6. Serve chilled or at room temperature.

Dopamine-Enhancing Breakfast Quesadilla

Ingredients:

- 2 whole grain tortillas

- 2 eggs, scrambled

- 1/4 cup black beans, drained and rinsed

- 1/4 cup diced tomatoes

- 1/4 cup shredded cheddar cheese

- Salsa and Greek yogurt for serving

Instructions:

1. Heat a skillet over medium heat.

2. Place one tortilla in the skillet and top with scrambled eggs, black beans, diced tomatoes, and shredded cheddar cheese.

3. Place the second tortilla on top.

4. Cook until the bottom tortilla is golden brown, then carefully flip and cook the other side until golden brown and the cheese is melted.

5. Slice into wedges and serve with salsa and Greek yogurt.

Dopamine-Boosting Breakfast Wrap

Ingredients:

- 1 whole grain wrap

- 2 tablespoons cream cheese

- 1/4 cup sliced strawberries

- 1/4 cup sliced bananas

- 1 tablespoon honey

- 1 tablespoon chopped almonds

Instructions:

1. Spread cream cheese evenly on the whole grain wrap.

2. Arrange sliced strawberries and bananas on top of the cream cheese.

3. Drizzle with honey and sprinkle with chopped almonds.

4. Roll up the wrap and slice

LUNCH RECIPES

Dopamine-Boosting Quinoa Salad

- Ingredients:

  - Quinoa, cooked

  - Spinach leaves

- Cherry tomatoes, halved

- Avocado, diced

- Almonds, chopped

- Olive oil

- Lemon juice

- Salt and pepper to taste

- Instructions:

1. In a large bowl, combine cooked quinoa, spinach leaves, cherry tomatoes, avocado, and chopped almonds.

2. Drizzle with olive oil and lemon juice.

3. Season with salt and pepper to taste. Toss gently to combine. Serve chilled.

Turkey and Avocado Wrap

- Ingredients:

- Whole wheat tortilla wraps

- Sliced turkey breast

- Avocado, mashed

- Baby spinach leaves

- Sliced red bell pepper

- Hummus (optional)

- Instructions:

1. Lay a tortilla wrap flat.

2. Spread mashed avocado on the tortilla.

3. Layer with sliced turkey breast, baby spinach leaves, sliced red bell pepper, and hummus if desired.

4. Roll tightly and slice into halves or quarters. Serve fresh.

Salmon and Quinoa Bowl

- Ingredients:

- Cooked quinoa

- Grilled or baked salmon fillet

- Steamed broccoli florets

- Sliced cucumbers

- Shredded carrots

- Lemon wedges

- Fresh dill (optional)

- Instructions:

1. Arrange cooked quinoa in bowls.

2. Top with grilled or baked salmon fillet, steamed broccoli florets, sliced cucumbers, and shredded carrots.

3. Garnish with lemon wedges and fresh dill if desired. Serve warm.

Dopamine-Boosting Lentil Soup

- Ingredients:

- Brown lentils, rinsed and drained

- Chopped onions

- Minced garlic

- Chopped carrots

- Chopped celery

- Vegetable or chicken broth

- Diced tomatoes

- Bay leaves

- Ground cumin

- Salt and pepper to taste

- Instructions:

1. In a large pot, sauté onions, garlic, carrots, and celery until softened.

2. Add lentils, diced tomatoes, bay leaves, ground cumin, and vegetable or chicken broth.

3. Bring to a boil, then reduce heat and simmer until lentils are tender.

4. Season with salt and pepper to taste. Serve hot.

Mediterranean Chickpea Salad

- Ingredients:

  - Canned chickpeas, rinsed and drained

  - Diced cucumbers

  - Diced tomatoes

  - Chopped red onions

  - Kalamata olives, sliced

  - Crumbled feta cheese

  - Chopped fresh parsley

  - Olive oil

  - Red wine vinegar

  - Dried oregano

  - Salt and pepper to taste

- Instructions:

1. In a large bowl, combine chickpeas, cucumbers, tomatoes, red onions, Kalamata olives, crumbled feta cheese, and chopped fresh parsley.

2. Drizzle with olive oil and red wine vinegar.

3. Sprinkle with dried oregano, salt, and pepper. Toss gently to combine. Serve chilled.

Spinach and Feta Stuffed Portobello Mushrooms

- Ingredients:

  - Large portobello mushrooms

  - Fresh spinach leaves

  - Crumbled feta cheese

  - Minced garlic

- Olive oil

- Balsamic glaze (optional)

- Salt and pepper to taste

- Instructions:

1. Preheat oven to 375°F (190°C).

2. Remove stems from portobello mushrooms and brush with olive oil.

3. In a skillet, sauté fresh spinach leaves with minced garlic until wilted.

4. Stuff portobello mushrooms with sautéed spinach and crumbled feta cheese.

5. Bake for 15-20 minutes until mushrooms are tender and cheese is melted.

6. Drizzle with balsamic glaze if desired. Season with salt and pepper. Serve warm.

Dopamine-Boosting Tofu Stir-Fry

- Ingredients:

- Extra-firm tofu, cubed

- Sliced bell peppers (assorted colors)

- Sliced mushrooms

- Broccoli florets

- Sliced carrots

- Minced ginger

- Minced garlic

- Low-sodium soy sauce

- Sesame oil

- Red pepper flakes (optional)

- Cooked brown rice or quinoa (for serving)

- Instructions:

1. In a wok or large skillet, heat sesame oil over medium-high heat.

2. Add cubed tofu and stir-fry until lightly browned.

3. Add sliced bell peppers, mushrooms, broccoli florets, and sliced carrots to the skillet.

4. Stir in minced ginger and garlic. Cook until vegetables are tender-crisp.

5. Drizzle with low-sodium soy sauce and sprinkle with red pepper flakes if desired.

6. Serve over cooked brown rice or quinoa.

Dopamine-Enhancing Chickpea Curry

- Ingredients:

  - Canned chickpeas, rinsed and drained

  - Chopped onions

  - Minced garlic

  - Diced tomatoes

- Coconut milk

- Curry powder

- Ground turmeric

- Ground cumin

- Ground coriander

- Red pepper flakes (optional)

- Fresh cilantro for garnish

- Cooked basmati rice (for serving)

- Instructions:

1. In a large skillet, sauté onions and garlic until translucent.

2. Add diced tomatoes, chickpeas, coconut milk, curry powder, ground turmeric, ground cumin, ground coriander, and red pepper flakes if desired.

3. Simmer for 15-20 minutes until flavors meld together and sauce thickens.

4. Garnish with fresh cilantro. Serve over cooked basmati rice.

9. Dopamine-Boosting Chicken Salad

  - Ingredients:

  - Cooked chicken breast, shredded or diced

    - Chopped celery

    - Diced apples

    - Dried cranberries

    - Chopped walnuts

    - Greek yogurt

    - Dijon mustard

    - Lemon juice

    - Honey

    - Salt and pepper to taste

  - Instructions:

1. In a large bowl, combine cooked chicken breast, chopped celery, diced apples, dried cranberries, and chopped walnuts.

2. In a separate bowl, whisk together Greek yogurt, Dijon mustard, lemon juice, honey, salt, and pepper to make

Certainly! Here are 50 lunch recipes designed to support dopamine nutrition, along with ingredients and instructions:

Dopamine-Boosting Quinoa Salad

- Ingredients:

  - Quinoa, cooked

  - Spinach leaves

  - Cherry tomatoes, halved

  - Avocado, diced

  - Almonds, chopped

  - Olive oil

- Lemon juice

- Salt and pepper to taste

- Instructions:

1. In a large bowl, combine cooked quinoa, spinach leaves, cherry tomatoes, avocado, and chopped almonds.

2. Drizzle with olive oil and lemon juice.

3. Season with salt and pepper to taste. Toss gently to combine. Serve chilled.

Turkey and Avocado Wrap

- Ingredients:

- Whole wheat tortilla wraps

- Sliced turkey breast

- Avocado, mashed

- Baby spinach leaves

- Sliced red bell pepper

- Hummus (optional)

- Instructions:

1. Lay a tortilla wrap flat.

2. Spread mashed avocado on the tortilla.

3. Layer with sliced turkey breast, baby spinach leaves, sliced red bell pepper, and hummus if desired.

4. Roll tightly and slice into halves or quarters. Serve fresh.

Salmon and Quinoa Bowl

- Ingredients:

  - Cooked quinoa

  - Grilled or baked salmon fillet

  - Steamed broccoli florets

  - Sliced cucumbers

  - Shredded carrots

- Lemon wedges

- Fresh dill (optional)

- Instructions:

1. Arrange cooked quinoa in bowls.

2. Top with grilled or baked salmon fillet, steamed broccoli florets, sliced cucumbers, and shredded carrots.

3. Garnish with lemon wedges and fresh dill if desired. Serve warm.

Dopamine-Boosting Lentil Soup

- Ingredients:

- Brown lentils, rinsed and drained

- Chopped onions

- Minced garlic

- Chopped carrots

- Chopped celery

- Vegetable or chicken broth

- Diced tomatoes

- Bay leaves

- Ground cumin

- Salt and pepper to taste

- Instructions:

1. In a large pot, sauté onions, garlic, carrots, and celery until softened.

2. Add lentils, diced tomatoes, bay leaves, ground cumin, and vegetable or chicken broth.

3. Bring to a boil, then reduce heat and simmer until lentils are tender.

4. Season with salt and pepper to taste. Serve hot.

Mediterranean Chickpea Salad

- Ingredients:

- Canned chickpeas, rinsed and drained

- Diced cucumbers

- Diced tomatoes

- Chopped red onions

- Kalamata olives, sliced

- Crumbled feta cheese

- Chopped fresh parsley

- Olive oil

- Red wine vinegar

- Dried oregano

- Salt and pepper to taste

- Instructions:

1. In a large bowl, combine chickpeas, cucumbers, tomatoes, red onions, Kalamata olives, crumbled feta cheese, and chopped fresh parsley.

2. Drizzle with olive oil and red wine vinegar.

3. Sprinkle with dried oregano, salt, and pepper. Toss gently to combine. Serve chilled.

Spinach and Feta Stuffed Portobello Mushrooms

- Ingredients:

  - Large portobello mushrooms

  - Fresh spinach leaves

  - Crumbled feta cheese

  - Minced garlic

  - Olive oil

  - Balsamic glaze (optional)

  - Salt and pepper to taste

- Instructions:

1. Preheat oven to 375°F (190°C).

2. Remove stems from portobello mushrooms and brush with olive oil.

3. In a skillet, sauté fresh spinach leaves with minced garlic until wilted.

4. Stuff portobello mushrooms with sautéed spinach and crumbled feta cheese.

5. Bake for 15-20 minutes until mushrooms are tender and cheese is melted.

6. Drizzle with balsamic glaze if desired. Season with salt and pepper. Serve warm.

Dopamine-Boosting Tofu Stir-Fry

- Ingredients:

  - Extra-firm tofu, cubed

  - Sliced bell peppers (assorted colors)

  - Sliced mushrooms

  - Broccoli florets

- Sliced carrots

- Minced ginger

- Minced garlic

- Low-sodium soy sauce

- Sesame oil

- Red pepper flakes (optional)

- Cooked brown rice or quinoa (for serving)

- Instructions:

1. In a wok or large skillet, heat sesame oil over medium-high heat.

2. Add cubed tofu and stir-fry until lightly browned.

3. Add sliced bell peppers, mushrooms, broccoli florets, and sliced carrots to the skillet.

4. Stir in minced ginger and garlic. Cook until vegetables are tender-crisp.

5. Drizzle with low-sodium soy sauce and sprinkle with red pepper flakes if desired.

6. Serve over cooked brown rice or quinoa.

Dopamine-Enhancing Chickpea Curry

- Ingredients:

  - Canned chickpeas, rinsed and drained

  - Chopped onions

  - Minced garlic

  - Diced tomatoes

  - Coconut milk

  - Curry powder

  - Ground turmeric

  - Ground cumin

- Ground coriander

- Red pepper flakes (optional)

- Fresh cilantro for garnish

- Cooked basmati rice (for serving)

- Instructions:

1. In a large skillet, sauté onions and garlic until translucent.

2. Add diced tomatoes, chickpeas, coconut milk, curry powder, ground turmeric, ground cumin, ground coriander, and red pepper flakes if desired.

3. Simmer for 15-20 minutes until flavors meld together and sauce thickens.

4. Garnish with fresh cilantro. Serve over cooked basmati rice.

Dopamine-Boosting Chicken Salad

- Ingredients:

- Cooked chicken breast, shredded or diced

- Chopped celery

- Diced apples

- Dried cranberries

- Chopped walnuts

- Greek yogurt

- Dijon mustard

- Lemon juice

- Honey

- Salt and pepper to taste

- Instructions:

1. In a large bowl, combine cooked chicken breast, chopped celery, diced apples, dried cranberries, and chopped walnuts.

2. In a separate bowl, whisk together Greek yogurt, Dijon mustard, lemon juice, honey, salt, and pepper to make

DINNER RECIPES

Grilled Salmon with Asparagus and Quinoa

- Ingredients:

  - Salmon fillets

  - Asparagus spears

  - Quinoa

  - Olive oil

  - Lemon

  - Salt and pepper to taste

- Instructions:

1. Marinate salmon fillets with olive oil, lemon juice, salt, and pepper.

2. Grill the salmon until cooked through.

3. Roast asparagus spears with olive oil, salt, and pepper.

4. Cook quinoa according to package instructions.

5. Serve grilled salmon with roasted asparagus and quinoa.

Stir-Fried Tofu with Broccoli and Brown Rice

- Ingredients:

  - Firm tofu, cubed

  - Broccoli florets

  - Brown rice

  - Soy sauce

  - Sesame oil

  - Garlic, minced

  - Ginger, grated

- Instructions:

1. Sauté tofu cubes until golden brown.

2. Stir in minced garlic and grated ginger.

3. Add broccoli florets and stir-fry until tender-crisp.

4. Season with soy sauce and sesame oil.

5. Serve over cooked brown rice.

Turkey Meatballs with Zucchini Noodles

- Ingredients:

  - Ground turkey

  - Zucchini

  - Tomato sauce

  - Garlic, minced

  - Onion, diced

  - Italian seasoning

- Instructions:

1. Mix ground turkey with minced garlic, diced onion, and Italian seasoning.

2. Form into meatballs and bake until cooked through.

3. Spiralize zucchini into noodles.

4. Sauté zucchini noodles with tomato sauce until heated through.

5. Serve turkey meatballs over zucchini noodles.

Chickpea and Vegetable Curry

- Ingredients:

  - Chickpcas

  - Mixed vegetables (e.g., bell peppers, carrots, peas)

  - Coconut milk

  - Curry paste or powder

  - Onion, diced

- Garlic, minced

- Basmati rice

- Instructions:

1. Sauté diced onion and minced garlic until softened.

2. Add mixed vegetables and chickpeas.

3. Stir in curry paste or powder and coconut milk.

4. Simmer until vegetables are tender.

5. Serve over cooked basmati rice.

Grilled Chicken with Roasted Vegetables

- Ingredients:

- Chicken breast

- Assorted vegetables (e.g., bell peppers, zucchini, carrots)

- Olive oil

- Balsamic vinegar

- Rosemary

- Salt and pepper to taste

- Instructions:

1. Marinate chicken breast in olive oil, balsamic vinegar, rosemary, salt, and pepper.

2. Grill chicken until cooked through.

3. Toss assorted vegetables with olive oil, salt, and pepper.

4. Roast vegetables until tender.

5. Serve grilled chicken with roasted vegetables.

Embracing the Dopamine Nutrition Lifestyle

Congratulations on completing your journey through "The Dopamine Nutrition Diet Cookbook." You've not only explored the fascinating connection between nutrition and dopamine but also discovered a wealth of delicious recipes and lifestyle strategies to support your overall well-being.

Reflecting on Your Journey

Take a moment to reflect on how far you've come. You've learned about the importance of dopamine in brain function and how nutrition plays a pivotal role in regulating its levels. By embracing the principles of the Dopamine Nutrition Diet, you've empowered yourself to make informed choices about the foods you eat and the way you nourish your body.

Continuing Dopamine-Supporting Practices

As you move forward, remember that the journey to optimal health is ongoing. Stay mindful of the foods you consume and how they impact your mood, energy levels, and overall vitality. Incorporate dopamine-boosting ingredients into your meals whenever possible, and savor each bite with gratitude and awareness.

Beyond the kitchen, prioritize other aspects of your lifestyle that contribute to dopamine balance. Engage in regular physical activity, practice stress-management techniques, and cultivate meaningful connections with others. Remember that a holistic approach to health encompasses not only what you eat but also how you live.

www.ingramcontent.com/pod-product-compliance
Lightning Source LLC
Chambersburg PA
CBHW050843260726
48660CB00006B/2405